MW00475349

Diabetes

Diabetes blackbook: Reverse diabetes forever with 25 superfoods

© **Copyright 2016 by Jasmin Lynch - All rights reserved.**

This document is geared towards providing exact and reliable information in regards to the topic and issue covered. The publication is sold with the idea that the publisher is not required to render accounting, officially permitted, or otherwise, qualified services. If advice is necessary, legal or professional, a practiced individual in the profession should be ordered.

- From a Declaration of Principles which was accepted and approved equally by a Committee of the American Bar Association and a Committee of Publishers and Associations.

In no way is it legal to reproduce, duplicate, or transmit any part of this document in either electronic means or in printed format. Recording of this publication is strictly prohibited and any storage of this document is not allowed unless with written permission from the publisher. All rights reserved.

The information provided herein is stated to be truthful and consistent, in that any liability, in terms of inattention or otherwise, by any usage or abuse of any policies, processes, or directions contained within is the solitary and utter responsibility of the recipient reader. Under no circumstances will any legal responsibility or blame be held against the publisher for any reparation, damages, or monetary loss due to the information herein, either directly or indirectly.

Respective authors own all copyrights not held by the publisher.

The information herein is offered for informational purposes solely, and is universal as so. The presentation of the information is without contract or any type of guarantee assurance.

The trademarks that are used are without any consent, and the publication of the trademark is without permission or backing by the trademark owner. All trademarks and brands within this book are for clarifying purposes only and are the owned by the owners themselves, not affiliated with this document.

Table of Contents:

Introduction

Let me extend my sincere delight that you have decided to download this eBook, *"Diabetes Black Book"*. I hope you find it rewarding and as enjoyable as I did in writing it.

This book includes proven strategies and steps on how you can reverse diabetes forever with just 25 super foods.

The number of fake promises and unclear information about how to lead with diabetes and to improve quality of life has been increasing more and more through many social networks. Be aware!

Here you can find a reliable source and important information about this disease; tips on how to manage with it; what is necessary to have a healthy and balanced diet and much more.

Moreover, you can learn delicious recipes made by ingredients that you should be sure to bring to your table.

I hope you enjoy reading this book!

Thanks again for downloading this book!

Chapter 1: What is diabetes?

Did you know that diabetes afflicts more than 380 million people around the world? Diabetes kills more people than Aids and breast cancer combined, one American every three minutes. Yes, this is an alarming statistic.

Let's understand its meaning first. Then we can discuss the role of insulin in our body, and if you might be at risk for it.

1.1 Definition:

Diabetes is a metabolism disorder, which causes high blood glucose (blood sugar).
It is a vital source of energy and the brain's source for fuel too.
If your body starts producing too much glucose, you'll have some serious health problems.

1.2 How to diagnose diabetes:

- **Prediabetes:**

Before developing diabetes, people almost have what is referred to as "**prediabetes**" –The levels of your blood sugar are higher than normal in prediabetes, but it is not high enough to actually be diagnosed as diabetes.

- **Type I and II:**

Chronic diabetes is divided in two groups: Type I and Type II.

Type I: It is generally diagnosed in children and young adults. In Type I diabetes, the body stops producing insulin, so a daily insulin shot is necessary.

Type II: When you have diabetes type II, your cells become resistant to insulin.

The problem is that the majority of people don't notice the signs or symptoms.

Here are a few signs that you should pay attention to:

- **Increased urination (Polyuria)** - The body in an effort to restore a normal blood sugar level, will try to eliminate the excess of sugar through urine. Then, you will feel a need to constantly go to the bathroom.
- **Increased thirst (Polydipsia)** - If you seem to be drinking a lot, but your thirst isn't quenched; then something might be wrong.
- **Increased of hunger (Polyphagia)** - If you are constantly feeling the urge to eat and you are never satisfied; this could be a sign of diabetes.
- **Fatigue** – Your body uses glucose for fuel, if you have a

lack of insulin you will become weakened. The lack of energy results in the sugar remaining in the blood instead of going into the cells. Inefficient energy can result in feelings of tiredness, mainly after meals.

- Pain or numbness in the feet and hands - High blood sugar can cause damage to the nerves and cause numbness in the hands and feet.

Chapter 2: Reversing Diabetes Naturally

Food has a great influence in treating diabetes. So if you eat properly, it is possible to reverse Type II and Type I diabetes naturally.

Below there is a list of foods you must ban from your menu to try to reverse diabetes.

- Refined sugar will cause the blood sugar to spike. Natural sweeteners such as raw honey or even maple syrup are better options, but these can still affect the blood sugar. The best option is to use **"stevia sweetener"**.

- Dried fruit, specially sweetened, contains higher levels of carbohydrates than natural fruit.

- Do not consume to much fruit juice (even if it is 100% natural)

- Sweetened beverages such as soda, powdered drinks, energy drinks and sports drinks must be avoided.

- Conventional or regular cow's milk ought to be eliminated mainly for type I diabetics. You can substitute it for **goat's milk**. Beware all other forms of dairy products, because in certain cases milk produced by the conventional dairy can damage the body and trigger an allergy to gluten. Buy dairy products that are raw and organic from animals raised in pastures.

- Grains (during the first 90 days), you'd better remove all grains. After this period, you could start introducing ancient grains in small quantities.

- Alcohol can increase glucose. Alcoholic beverages such as Beer and other sweet liquors should be avoided. These are very high in carbohydrates.

- GMO corn, soy, canola and hydrogenated oils may promote diabetes, so they are best to be avoided.

Chapter 3: What should you drink?

When you are a diabetic, everybody worries about the food you eat, but remember that the beverages you drink are going to affect your blood sugar as well.

Raw juicing, vegetables juicing and green juices are very powerful, mainly for people fighting diabetes, obesity, heart disease, cancer, or any other degenerative disease. Juicing can be very nutritious, but you have to drink greener vegetables/ grasses and avoid drinking too much fruit juices.

Green juices and green smoothies stimulate the production of hemoglobin and also Chlorophyll which repairs tissue and is very important in helping to remove toxins from our body.

Below there are some beverages you can drink without guilt.

Water: It is the top beverage. You can drink anytime. But if you don't want to drink just water, try to spice up adding some berries, lime or lemons in it. Remember: no sugar or syrup in it!

Green tea: it regulates glucose levels in the body; it can also prevent the progression of type I diabetes and reduce blood sugar levels in type II diabetes.

Black tea: it helps people by slowing glucose absorption and it may protect against diabetes by mimicking the effects of insulin in the body.

Kale: it is low in carbohydrates, contains some proteins, and provides a wide assortment of vitamins and minerals.

**Coffee: moderate coffee consumption – around 4 cups a day – can contribute to water intake but be cautious what you put in your coffee. Even creamers or fat milk can increase calories and sugar intake.

*If you have heart disease or high blood pressure, talk to your doctor about caffeine consumption!

Note: ** Coffee is a little controversial, some doctors ban it completely and others assure that coffee, if consume moderately, can help reverse diabetes.

Juice Recipes that help reversing Type II Diabetes:

1. Spinach Celery Juice

Ingredients:

- 3 Fistfuls of spinach
- 2 celery stalks with leaves

- 1 carrot

- 1 green apple

- 1 cucumber (if desired)

Instructions:

1. Wash and peel the carrot and green apple. Then remove the apple seeds.
2. Juice the carrot and green apple together with spinach and celery.

2. Watercress, Tomatoes and Parsley Juice

This is a healthy juicing recipe effective in helping to prevent heart disease and strokes. It can be found in daily consumption of apple juice or in green apple juices helping lower cholesterol levels.

Ingredients:

- 6 sprigs of watercress
- 1 fistful of parsley

- 2 tomatoes

- 2 apples

Instructions:

1. Slice apples in wedges and remove both the core and the seed.
2. Put everything in the blender and mix.

Chapter 4: Fruits that reverse diabetes:

Fruits are organized into 5 categories: pomes, drupes, berries, citrus and melons.

Pomes – these fruits are an excellent source of vitamins and fiber.
Examples: apples and pears

Drupes – they supply both ß-carotene and vitamin C, with some potassium and fiber.
Examples: Apricots, peaches, nectarines, plums, and cherries.

Berries – they are good antioxidants and fiber.
Examples: grapes, dates, raspberries, strawberries, blueberries, eggplants, tomatoes, peppers, and several other fruits.

Citrus – they have high vitamin C and flavonoids. Grapes and oranges also contain a good amount of fiber.
Example: oranges, tangerines, grapefruits, lemons, and limes.

Melons – melons are a good source of vitamin C; however, while orange-fleshed melons are rich in ß-carotene, red watermelons are rich in lycopede.

This fruit group is equally divided into 2 classes of melons: muskmelons and watermelons. There are several different types of watermelons. The muskmelon class includes cantaloupe, casaba, honeydew and several others.

Tropical fruit – they have unique texture and flavors.

- **Lowest in Sugar**

  Lemon/ Lime
  Rhubarb
  Raspberries
  Blackberries
  Cranberries

- **Low to Medium In Sugar**

  Casaba Melon
  Strawberries
  Papaya
  Nectarines
  Peaches
  Blueberries
  Honeydew Melons
  Cantaloupes
  Apples
  Apricot
  Guavas
  Grapefruit

- **Fairly High In Sugar**

  Plums
  Oranges
  Kiwifruit
  Pears
  Pineapple
  Watermelon

- **Very High in Sugar**

  Tangerines
  Cherries

Grapes
Pomegranates
Mangos
Figs
Bananas
Dried Fruit (dates, raisins, prunes, dried apricot, etc.)

Chapter 5: Useful tips

Adding a snack in your meal plan

It is a great way to add vitamins, fiber and minerals. But keep track of the carbohydrates you eat because it is important for balancing your blood sugar.

Below there are some nutritious snack options (~ 5 g of carbohydrate):

- 1 cup air popped popcorn
- 12-15 roasted or raw, unsalted almonds
- ½ cup of low-fat cottage cheese
- ¼ of a small avocado
- 1 low-fat string cheese
- 5 baby carrots with only one tablespoon peanut butter

Meal preparation

- Vegetables should be eaten fresh, lightly steamed, grilled or roasted.

- When they are not fresh, opt for the frozen vegetables and avoid eating canned ones.

- Pickles and sauerkraut are ok.

- Avoid bringing the vegetable to a boiling point.

- Avoid cooking them with cheese, butter, or sauce.

Diabetes meal plan

Having a diabetes meal plan is important because it tells you the quantity and what foods you can eat at meals and snack times.

It must include:

1. The plate method;

2. Carbohydrate counting;

3. Glycemic index

Your meal plan will help you improve blood glucose, blood pressure and cholesterol.

Ask Yourself, what is a healthy diet?

A healthy diet is the way someone eats which reduces risk for complications such as stroke or heart diseases.

Prefer the food rich in vitamins, mineral and fiber.

It must include eating a wide diversity of foods including:

- fruits

- vegetables
- non-fat dairy products

- Whole grains

- beans

- lean meats

- poultry

- fish

Chapter 6: A List of 25 Superfoods

This chapter provides a list of 25 superfoods, their description and how they can help you reverse diabetes.

Food description and its benefits:

1. **Green vegetables** are the important foods for you to focus on for diabetes prevention and reversal. A great leaf green intake can decrease in 14% the risk of type II diabetes. Its daily consumption decreases this risk in 9%.
    Vegetables are rich in fiber and you can have a cup of each vegetable at one time; vegetables are extremely low in carbohydrates.

    The best vegetables for diabetes are:

    - Artichokes
    - Asparagus

    - Bamboo shoots

    - Bean sprouts

    - Broccoli

    - Brussels sprouts

    - Cabbage

    - Carrot

    - Cauliflower

    - Celery

    - Chilies

    - Cucumbers

- Greens (Kale, collard, mustard and turnip)

- Mushrooms

- Parsley

- Romaine lettuce

- Spinach

- Tomatoes

- Turnip

- Water cress

- Zucchini

Avoid these vegetables or just eat them in smaller quantities:

- Corn
- Beets
- Sweet Potatoes

- potatoes

- Tapioca

- Yam

2. **Non-starchy vegetables**: they are essential components of a diabetes prevention or reversal diet. They have almost no effect on blood sugar, rich in fiber and phytochemicals. Mushrooms, onions, garlic, eggplant, peppers, etc ... are good examples of non-starchy vegetables.

3. **Allium:** it is often used to add some flavor to other foods, but can be eaten by themselves too. Onions, garlic, leeks, scallions, chives, and shallots are allium

vegetables. Allium vegetables boost immunity, diminish inflammation, and fight off disease.

4. **Nuts:** they are low in carbohydrates, high in proteins and fiber and rich in minerals (potassium). They also contain a large amount of unsaturated fat, which is good for cholesterol.
   * Nuts can be very caloric, so keep your unsalted portion in one serving.
   One serving is about ¼ of a cup.

5. **Complex Carbohydrates:** they contain fiber, are digested more slowly than simple carbohydrates, so glucose don't rise as high.

   Good examples of complex carbohydrates are the following:

   - Brown rice, oatmeal, whole-wheat pasta, whole grains, high fiber cereals, etc.
   - Some vegetables like broccoli, corn and legumes (kidney beans, chick peas), etc.

6. **Quinoa:** It is a grain, which is naturally gluten free and rich in fiber and protein.
   *It contains smaller amounts of carbohydrate than other starches per serving.

7. **Extra Virgin Olive Oil:** it helps you lose weight, stabilizes blood sugar levels, it can help prevent diabetes and limit the complications from it.

8. **Fresh fruit:** they are rich in fiber and antioxidants. Low sugar fruits like berries, kiwi, orange, and melon can minimize glycemic effects and they are ideal for diabetes.

9. **Salmon, tuna, trout, mackerel, and sardines:** they are rich in Omega 3.

10. **Beans**: they can prevent diabetes or they can minimize its effects because Beans help to regulate the blood glucose and insulin levels. Also, beans help to reduce cholesterol levels while offering anti-oxidant properties.

    Red beans offers the highest anti-oxidant levels; they are trailed by black beans.

11. **Coconut oil:** its medium chain of fatty acids are immediately converted to be available as energy.

12. **Seaweed, "wakame", and brown seaweed:** it helps in the process of weight lost; it helps to promote the fat-burning proteins and help avoid diabetes.

13. **Cinnamon** is effective against diabetes; it mends the blood sugar regulation by considerably increasing the glucose metabolism.

14. **White eggs:** amino acids found in white eggs stimulate "wake-you-up" brain cells, called orexin cells. It is also a way to energize.

15. **Dark chocolate** lowers your risk of insulin resistance. *If must be raw, unprocessed without any refined sugar.

16. **Baking Chocolate and Cocoa powder**

17. **Salmon:** it's rich in Omega 3 – 6, it protects your heart

18. **Apples:** reduce the symptoms of diabetes and keep blood sugar steady. It is also rich in fiber what helps your digestion and keeps you more fit. Green apples contain malic acid, which helps in lowering your sugar level.

19. **Almonds:** lowers the risk of a coronary heart disease.

20. **Celery:** is rich in **magnesium** and **potassium.** It includes minerals and sodium to help regulate blood pressure.

21. **Carrots:** are rich in the antioxidant ß-carotene, vitamin A, B, C and K, dietary fiber and magnesium. They are a great low carbohydrate, a good blood regulator and they are excellent for helping eye problems in diabetics.

22. **Tomatoes:** contain the powerful antioxidant – lycopene, vitamin A, C, K, phosphorus, calcium, potassium, foliate and dietary fiber. All tomato-based products are extremely low in carbohydrates.

23. **Spinach:** contains beta-carotene, **calcium**, vitamins A and C that provides multiple health benefits.

24. **Squash and zucchini:** it contains vitamin A, B and C, iron, calcium, dietary fiber, potassium and magnesium. Add color to your stir-fry, steam or grill for allow-carbohydrate side dish.

25. **Watercress**: it is packed full of beta carotene and antioxidants which are crucial in lessening the risk of heart disease, cataracts and some types of cancers.

This list of food is only an example, there are many other ones if combined correctly they can bring you infinite benefits.

Chapter 7: Delicious foods and easy recipes

1. **Good snacks:**

- 2 egg whites (hard boiled) with ¼ c. ricotta cheese (part-skim) and some diced red pepper mixture on a slice of whole wheat bread (15 grams of carbs per slice).

- 1 small apple (~4oz) with 1 tbsp of all natural peanut butter, cashew butter, almond butter or sun butter.

- ½c. of frozen peaches (you can warm these in the microwave) mixed with 6oz of low –fat vanilla Greek yogurt with 2 teaspoons of ground flaxseed.

2. **High Protein, high fiber, 30g Carbohydrate breakfast:**

- 3 scrambled egg whites plus 1 whole egg, with ½ c. of cooked spinach; ¼ c. of shredded low-fat cheese and 2 slices of whole grain bread (100% whole rye, wheat or oat bread).

- 1 non-fat Greek yogurt can be mixed with a ½ c. low-fat cottage cheese, ¾c. of blueberries and 2 tablespoons of chopped almonds.

- 1 English muffin ,whole grain, with 2 tbsp of peanut butter and a few sliced strawberries and 2 slices of low-sodium turkey.

- ½ c. of cooked oatmeal, with ½ c. sliced peaches, with 2 hard-boiled egg whites and 1 tbsp of ground flaxseed.

3. **Tuna Spinach Salad:**

   1. Omit the mayonnaise and mix tuna with 2 tablespoons of hummus.

   2. Mix together spinach, carrots, cucumber and other non-starchy vegetables.

   3. Add ½ cup beans (rinse in water first if it is canned).

   4. Mix vinegar with one-tbsp. of olive oil for a dressing.

      *You can add fresh garlic and hot pepper to the dressing.

4. **Roasted Peppers and Onion Chicken Burger:**

   1. Grill your burger or bake it in an oven.

   2. Place a burger patty between a whole grain bun or just avoid using the bun all together to lower the amount of carbohydrates. Then place your burger on the top of the green salad with ½ c. of black beans and a ¼ c. of shredded low-fat mozzarella cheese.

5. **Open Faced Roasted Turkey Sandwich with Sweet Potato Fries:**

Put a slice of turkey tenderloin on a single slice of whole grain bread, top sautéed spinach and a fistful of sweet potato fries (leftover from last night's meal).

6. Grilled Chicken with Corn Creamy

Serves: 4

Serving Size: 1 half of a breast and 1/3 c. of creamy corn mixture

Ingredients:

- 2 tblps Olive oil
- 1 tsp smoked paprika
- 3 ears of corn, husks and silks removed
- 4 skinless, boneless chicken breast halves (1 to 1-1/4 pounds total)
- 1/4 tsp salt
- 1/8 tsp black pepper
- 1/3c. light sour cream
- Fat-free milk
- 1/4 c. Basil, shredded fresh

Instructions:

1. In a small size bowl combine the olive oil and paprika. Then brush the corn and chicken with the oil mixture. Sprinkle with pepper and salt.
2. For a charcoal grill, you can place the corn and chicken on rack directly over medium coals. Then grill, uncovered, for 12 -15 minutes or until the chicken is completely done and no longer pinkish at about 170 degrees F, turn it only once.

(If using a gas grill, preheat it. Then reduce the heat to medium. Place the corn and chicken on the grill rack over the heat. Cover and grill as instructed for the charcoal grill above.)

3. Place one ear of corn on a cutting board with the pointed tip down. Hold corn securely at stem end to hold it in place, while using a sharp knife to cut corn from the cob. Leave some of the corn in planks; then rotate the cob as needed in order to cut the corn off all sides.
4. Repeat the process with the remaining ears of corn. (A kitchen towel can be used to grip, if necessary.) Once this is done, transfer the corn to a bowl; then stir in the sour cream. Carefully, stir in some milk to the desired creaminess you would like. Slice chicken breasts.

7. Sprinkle with shredded basil

7. Coconut Crust Pizza

Total Time: 25-30 minutes
Serves: 1 pizza

Preheat oven to 350 degrees Fahrenheit.
Time: 20 minutes

Ingredients:
- ¼ cup + 2 tablespoon coconut flour
- ¼ coconut oil

- 3 eggs

- 1 tablespoon honey

- 1 tablespoon baking powder

- ¼ tablespoon sea salt

Instructions:
1. Line a pizza sheet with parchment paper.
2. In a bowl, mix together the wet ingredients and the dry ingredients in another.
3. Combine the wet and dry ingredients.
4. Roll batter onto parchment paper until about ½-¾ in thick
5. Take the crust out and top with favorite ingredients.
6. After placing back in to the oven, bake it for about 2-3 more minutes or just until the cheese has melted.

8. Carrot Broccoli Soup
Total Time: 35 minutes
Serves: 4 servings

Ingredients:

- 1 medium onion (chopped)
- 2 medium carrots (chopped)
- 1 tablespoon butter
- 3 cups of fresh broccoli florets
- 2 celery ribs (chopped)
- 3 cups of fat-free milk (divided)

- ¾ teaspoon of salt

- ½ teaspoon of dried thyme

- ⅛ Teaspoon of pepper

- 3 tablespoons all-purpose flour

Instructions:

1. Spray a large saucepan with cooking spray; then cook the carrots, onion, and celery in butter for 3 minutes.
2. Add broccoli; cool 3 minutes longer.

3. Stir in 2¾ c. of milk, thyme, salt and pepper.

4. Bring the mixture to a boil. Reduce heat; cover and simmer until the vegetables are done for about 5-10 minutes.

5. Combine the flour and the remaining milk until smooth; gradually stirring it into the soup. Bringing back to a boil; cook for about 2 minutes longer or until thickened.

9. Walnut Crusted Salmon:

Total Time: 35 minutes
Serves: 4 servings

Preheat oven to 400°

Ingredients:
- 4 salmon fillets (4 ounces each)
- 4 teaspoons honey

- 4 teaspoons Dijon mustard

- 2 slices whole wheat bread, torn into crumb size

- 3 tablespoons finely chopped walnuts

- 2 teaspoons canola oil

- 1/2 teaspoon dried thyme

Instructions:

1. Place salmon on a baking sheet coated with cooking spray.

2. Mix honey and mustard; brush it over salmon.

3. Place bread in a food processor; pulse until coarse crumbs form.

4. Transfer to a small bowl. Then stir in the walnuts, oil and thyme; press onto salmon.

5. Bake 12-15 minutes or until topping is lightly browned and the fish just begins to flake easily with a fork.

10. **Orange Chicken**

Total Time: 35 minutes

Serves: 5 servings

Ingredients:

1 ¼ Lbs. Chicken breasts, Boneless, skinless
2 Tbsp. Cornstarch
2 Tbsp. Flour
2 Tbsp. Vegetable oil
½ Cup Orange juice, Fresh
½ Cup Water

2 Tbsp. Soy sauce, Reduced-sodium
1 Tbsp. Ginger, Fresh grated
1 tsp. Sugar
¼ tsp. ground coriander
¼ tsp. black or white pepper, freshly ground
½ cup Scallions, thinly sliced
1 Tbsp. Sesame seeds, toasted
2 tsp. Orange zest, fresh
¼-½ tsp. Red chili flakes

Instructions:

1. Cut the chicken into 1-inch size cubes. In a large bowl, combine the cornstarch and the flour. Then add the chicken. Toss to coat the chicken with the flour mixture.

2. In a large skillet, heat the oil over medium-high heat. Adding the chicken and stir-fry for about 6 to 7 minutes, or until the chicken is golden browned and cooked through. The chicken can be removed from the skillet and set aside to drain.

3. Drain the excess grease from the skillet. Then add the water, orange juice, soy sauce, ginger, sugar, coriander, and the pepper. Bring this mixture to the boiling point, then lower the heat. Simmering for 5 to 6 minutes, or until slightly thickened.

4. Once the sauce is thickened, place the chicken into the sauce and simmer this for about 2 minutes. Add in the scallions, orange zest, sesame seeds, and the chili flakes. Serve immediately.

11. Veggie Sausage Cheddar Frittata

Total Time: 15 minutes

Serves: 4 servings

Ingredients:

- 1 green bell pepper, chopped

- 4 (1.3-ounce) frozen vegetable protein sausage patties, thawed and crumbled

- Cooking spray
- 1 (8-ounce) package presliced mushrooms

- 1 cup egg substitute

- 1/8 teaspoon salt

- 1/4 cup fat-free half-and-half

- 1/8 teaspoon Black pepper, freshly ground

- 1/2 cup (2 ounces) Cheddar cheese, shredded reduced-fat sharp

Instructions:

1. Preheat broiler.

2. Over medium-high heat, place your 12-inch ovenproof nonstick skillet.

3. Coat skillet with your choice of cooking spray. Add in the chopped bell pepper and the mushrooms; sauté 3 minutes.

4. Add in the sausage, pepper, and salt; then reduce the heat to a medium-low heat. Cook for 1 minute.

5. Combine the egg substitute and the half-and-half; carefully pour this mixture over sausage mixture.

6. Cover and cook 6 minutes. (It will be somewhat moist on top.)

7. Sprinkle with cheese.

8. Broil for 1 to 2 minutes or until the cheese melts.

9. Cut this into 8 wedges

12. **Veggie Tostadas**

Total Time: 30 minutes

Serves: 4 servings

Ingredients:

- 2 cups sliced mushrooms

- 1 large red bell pepper, chopped

- 2 small zucchini, sliced

- 4 BASIC TOSTADAS

- Cooking spray

Preparation
1. Coat a medium nonstick skillet with the cooking spray on medium heat until it is hot.
2. Add in the zucchini, mushrooms, and bell pepper to pan.
3. Sautée this for 3 to 5 minutes or until the vegetables are tender.
4. Now Spoon about 3/4 cup of the vegetable mixture over the black bean mixture on each of the tostadas.
5. Top this with the lettuce, salsa, and then the cheese.

13. Snapper with a Tomato-Caper Topping

Total Time: 20 minutes

Serves: 4

Ingredients:

- 2 cups grape tomatões, halved
- 2 tablespoons lemon juice (about 1 lemon) fresh

- 2 tablespoons capers, drained

- 2 teaspoons olive oil

- 2 tablespoons chopped fresh parsley

- 1 1/2 teaspoons dried basil or 1 tablespoon fresh basil, shredded reduced-fat sharp

- 1/4 teaspoon salt

- 1/8 teaspoon red pepper, crushed (optional)

- 4 (6-ounce) Red snapper or grouper fillets (each fillets should be about 3/4 inch thick)

- Cooking spray

- 1 teaspoon paprika

- 1 Lemon, cut into 4 wedges

Instructions:

1. Mix the first 6 ingredients and crushed red pepper, set aside.

2. Place the grouper or snapper fillets on a broiler pan that has been lined with aluminum foil; coat the foil with the cooking spray. Sprinkle the fillets with the paprika; coat with cooking spray.

3. Bake for about 10 minutes at 450°

4. Top fillets with tomato mixture; then bake about 5 minutes or until the fish flakes easily when it is tested with a fork.

5. Sprinkle with the parsley, and serve it with lemon wedges.

14. Seared Chicken with Avocados

- 4 (4-ounce) skinless, boneless chicken breast halves

- 1 ½ teaspoons blackened seasoning
- 1 teaspoon Olive oil

- 1 diced peeled avocado

- 1 jalapeño pepper, seeded, finely chopped

- 2 tablespoons chopped fresh cilantro

- 2 tablespoons fresh lime juice (about 1 lime)

- 1 lime, cut into fourths

- 1/4 teaspoon salt

Instructions:

1. Sprinkle the seasoning on both sides of the chicken.

2. In a large nonstick skillet, heat the Olive oil over high heat. Add the chicken to the pan with the smooth side down; cook this 1 minute or until it is seared.

3. Reduce to medium heat; cook for 3 minutes on each side or until it is lightly browned.

4. Combine the avocado, three-fourths of the lime's juice, pepper, cilantro, and salt. Squeeze one-fourth of the lime over each piece of chicken before serving. Serve this with the avocado mixture.

15. Grilled Salmon:
Total Time: 20 minutes

Ingredients:
- Salmon
- Salt

Instructions:
1. Sprinkle salt on the salmon
2. Grill or broil it.

16. Mediterranean Stuffed Tomatoes:

Ingredients:
- 2 large tomatões

- 1/4 cup (1 ounce) goat cheese, crumbled

- 1/2 cup packaged garlic croutons

- 1/4 cup kalamata olives, sliced pitted

- 2 tablespoons thyme or basil, chopped fresh

- 2 tablespoons vinaigrette, reduced-fat or Italian salad dressing

Instructions:

1. Preheat broiler.

2. Cut the tomatoes crosswise in half. Using your fingers to push out and then discard the seeds. Using a paring knife to cut out the pulp, leave 2 shells.

3. Chop the pulp, and transfer it to a medium bowl. Place the hollowed out tomatoes with the cut sides down, onto a paper towel; drain them for about 5 minutes.

4. Add croutons, dressing, olives, goat cheese, and thyme or basil to pulp; mix this well. Mound up the mixture into hollowed tomatoes.

5. Place the tomatoes on a baking sheet or a broiler pan. Broil tomatoes 4-5 inches from the heat until hot and the cheese has melted (about 5 minutes). Serve it right away!

Desserts:

1. Chocolate-Caramel Coconut Flour Brownies

Total Time: 35 minutes
Serves: 9

Preheat oven to 350 degrees Fahrenheit.
Time: 25-30 minutes

Ingredients:

- 1 1/4 cup cacao powder

- 4 eggs

- 1/4 cup coconut flour
- 1 teaspoon sea salt

- 1 teaspoon baking soda

- 1/2 cup honey

- 1 tbsp. vanilla extract

- 1/4 cup coconut sugar

- 1/3 cup dark chocolate chips

- 1/3 cup coconut oil

- 1 homemade caramel recipe

Instructions:

1. Mix dry ingredients in one bowl and wet ingredients in a second bowl.
2. Combine both mixtures and stir until all ingredients are incorporated together.

3. Pour the mixture into a greased 8x8 pan.

4. Top with chocolate chips and/or nuts if desired.

5. Let cool and then drizzle with caramel sauce.

2. Coconut Flour Chocolate Chunk Bars

Serves: 16

Preheat oven to 350 degrees Fahrenheit.
Time: 20-22 minutes

Ingredients:

- ¼ cup melted coconut oil
- 2 teaspoons vanilla extract
- 1/3 cup agave nectar, honey, or maple syrup
- 2 eggs, beaten slightly
- ½ cup coconut flour
- ¼ cup almond milk, unsweetened
- ¼ teaspoon salt
- ½ teaspoon baking soda
- 1/2 cup coconut flakes, optional
- 3 oz. your favorite dairy free dark chocolate bar, coarsely chopped

Instructions:

1. Spray a 8x8 inch baking pan with nonstick cooking spray.
2. Whisk together honey, coconut oil, eggs, vanilla, and almond milk in a large bowl. Whisk together

baking soda, coconut flour, and salt in a separate medium bowl.

3. Add the dry ingredients to the wet ingredients. Mix until slightly combined and the batter is smooth.

4. Fold in the chopped chocolate, reserving a few tablespoons for sprinkling on top for garnish if desired.

5. Bake for about 22-25 minutes or until the edges are golden brown and the knife comes out with only a few crumbs attached to it.

6. The batter could appear like it is not completely cooked, but it will be. DO NOT OVERBAKE. This will result in the bars drying out and no one likes that!

7. Cut into 16 squares.

3. Apples with cinnamon:

1. Slice the apple and sprinkle some cinnamon.

2. Take to the microwave for about 2 minutes.

4. Applesauce Pancake:

Ingredients:

- 1 cup all-purpose flour
- 1 teaspoon baking soda
- 2 tablespoons toasted wheat germ
- 1/8 teaspoon salt

- 1/4 cup unsweetened applesauce

- 1 cup nonfat buttermilk

- 1 large egg, lightly beaten

- 2 teaspoons vegetable oil

- Cooking spray

- Fresh fruit slices (optional)

- Sugar-free maple syrup (optional)

Instructions:

1. Combine the first 4 ingredients in a medium size bowl; next make a well in the center of the mixture.

2. Combine the buttermilk and next 3 ingredients. Add the buttermilk mixture into the dry ingredients. Stirring this until dry ingredients are completely moistened.

3. Heat the nonstick griddle or a nonstick skillet that is coated with the cooking spray over a medium heat.

4. For each pancake, pour a 1/4 cup batter onto the hot griddle, spreading it to a 5-inch circle.

5. Continue to cook pancakes until the tops are covered with bubbles and edges look slightly cooked; then turn pancakes, and cook other side.

6. Serve pancakes with maple syrup and fresh fruit, if desired (the syrup and the fruit not included in the recipe).

Tip: One tablespoon of a sugar-free maple syrup has about 8 calories and 3 grams of carbohydrate.

5. Honey Grapefruit with Bananas

Ingredients:

- 1 (24-ounce) jar red grapefruit sections (about 2 cups), refrigerated
- 1 tablespoon fresh chopped mint
- 1 cup sliced banana (about 1)
- 1 tablespoon honey

Instructions:

1. Drain the grapefruit sections, reserve 1/4 cup juice.
2. Combine grapefruit sections, juice, and remaining ingredients in a medium bowl. Then toss gently to well coat. Serve it immediately, or cover and chill.

Note: you can substitute honey for stevia.

6. Fresh Berries with Maple Cream

Ingredients:

- 3/4 cup fat-free sour cream
- 1 cup fresh blueberries
- 1/4 cup maple syrup
- 1 1/2 cups fresh raspberries

Instructions:

1. Combine the sour cream and the maple syrup in a small bowl; stir this with a whisk.

2. Combine the berries, and spoon mixture into dessert dishes; then pour maple cream over berries.

7. Cantaloupe Sherbet

Ingredients:

- 1 large ripe cantaloupe, peeled and finely chopped (about 5 cups)
- 2 tablespoons lemon juice
- 1/3 cup "measures-like-sugar" calorie-free sweetener
- 2 teaspoons unflavored gelatin
- 1 (8-ounce) carton vanilla fat-free yogurt sweetened with aspartame
- 1/4 cup cold water
- Cantaloupe wedge (optional)

Instructions:

1. Combine the lemon juice, cantaloupe, and sweetener in a blender or a food processor; process until smooth. Transfer the mixture to a medium bowl.

2. Sprinkle the gelatin over cold water in a small saucepan; let this stand for 1 minute. Then Cook over low heat, stirring it until gelatin dissolves for about 4 minutes.

3. Add to the cantaloupe mixture, stirring it well. Add the yogurt, stirring until it is smooth.

4. Pour the mixture into an 8-inch square pan; freeze it until almost firm.

5. Transfer the mixture to a large bowl; beat with a mixer at high speed until it is fluffy. Spoon mixture back into the pan; then freeze until it is firm.

6. Scoop it into 5 individual serving dishes in order to serve. Garnish each serving with a cantaloupe wedge, optional (cantaloupe wedge not included in recipe).

8. Apple – Cinnamon Granola

Ingredients:

- 1 cup Cheerios or a oat cereal, whole-grain toasted
- 3 cups regular oats
- 2 teaspoons ground cinnamon
- 1/3 cup oat bran
- 1/3 cup walnuts, finely chopped
- 1/4 teaspoon ground cardamom
- 1/3 cup applesauce
- 2 tablespoons butter
- 1/4 cup honey
- 2 tablespoons brown sugar
- 1 cup chopped dried apple

- Cooking spray

Instructions:

Preheat the oven to 250°.

1. Combine the first 6 ingredients in a large bowl, stirring well to combine.

2. Melt 2 tablespoons of butter in a medium saucepan over medium heat.

3. Add 1/3 cup applesauce, brown sugar and honey to pan, and bring mix to a boil.

4. Cook mixture for 1 minute, stirring it frequently.

5. Pour the applesauce mixture over the oat mixture, stirring to coat.

6. Spread the mixture in an even layer on a jelly-roll pan that has been coated with cooking spray.

7. Bake in oven at 250° for 1 ½ hour, stirring every 30 minutes.

8. Allow this to cool completely. Then stir in chopped apple.

9. Morning Glory Muffins

Preheat oven to 350°.

Ingredients:

- Cooking spray
- 1/2 cup all-purpose flour (about 2 1/4 ounces)
- 1 cup whole wheat flour (about 4 3/4 ounces)
- 1 cup regular oats
- 1 tablespoon wheat bran
- 3/4 cup packed brown sugar
- 2 teaspoons baking soda
- 1/4 teaspoon salt
- 1 cup mashed ripe banana (about 2)
- 1 cup plain fat-free yogurt
- 1 large egg
- 3/4 cup chopped walnuts
- 1 cup chopped pitted dates
- 1/2 cup chopped dried pineapple
- 3 tablespoons ground flaxseed (about 2 tablespoons whole)

Instructions:

1. Place the 18 muffin cups liners in the muffin cups; coat the liners with cooking spray.

2. Lightly spoon the flours into dry measuring cups, and level it with a knife.

3. Combine flours and the next 5 ingredients (through salt) in a large bowl; stir with a whisk.

4. Next make a well in the center of the mixture.

5. Combine the banana, yogurt, and egg; adding to the flour mixture, stirring just until moisten.

6. Fold in the walnuts, dates, and pineapple.

7. Spoon the batter into the prepared muffin cups.

8. Sprinkle it evenly with the flaxseed.

9. Bake in the oven at 350° for approximately 20 minutes or until muffins spring back when touched lightly in the center.

10. Remove the muffins from the pans immediately; cool them on a wire rack.

Conclusion:

Thank you again for downloading this book!

I hope this book was able to help you to understand the importance of food and its role to reverse diabetes.

The next step is to make a meal plan and try delicious and easy recipes, which will help you, reverse diabetes naturally.

Finally, if you enjoyed this book, then I'd like to ask you for a favor, would you be kind enough to leave a review for this book on Amazon? It'd be greatly appreciated!

Thank you and good luck!

49377014R00030

Made in the USA
San Bernardino, CA
22 May 2017